This book is dedicated to my late Grandfathers, Kenneth England, who passed away in 1993 and Ray Lewis who passed away in 1992, both aged 70. Despite their respective health issues their determination and tenacity have inspired me to conquer my own issues.

I also want to mention my late aunties Penny England and Margaret Davis, who sadly lost their long fought battles with Lupus and Cancer respectively. They never complained and lived life to the full.

How I'm beating Psoriatic Arthritis.

Contents

Foreword

I am a 37 year old Engineer, husband and father of 2 girls aged 15 and 3. Life has never been straight forward for me, I have made a few poor decisions which have been character building at the very least.

Up until my late twenties I was physically fit, able bodied and took life for granted.

Reality hit me head on when a series of adversities struck, the sort of problems that would have probably sent most people over the edge. But after all the setbacks I'm still smiling, and coming out on top!

This book will take you through my story, from the time when I developed the first symptoms of Psoriatic Arthritis (Psa) aged 30, through the struggles that I faced, my diagnosis, reactions to treatment and my eventual transition from being a bit of a 'couch potato' to cycling 410 miles in 4 days for charity in 2012.

I do not want to preach about how great I may think I am or that you should do what I do, but I hope to tell my story and convey how the lessons I've learned could help or inspire you.

More so, I do not want to judge or make comparisons. Everyone copes with pain and stress in different ways and all cases of arthritis are unique to the sufferer.

This book is based purely on my own experiences and opinions. Please take what you want to from it but I offer no guarantees or promises.

I sincerely hope that you enjoy reading this book and that it helps to add value and enjoyment to your life.

<u>There is life after Arthritis.</u>

Chapter 1 – Life before Psa.

I want to start here because this period in my life was a real challenge and lead to problems which may have triggered Psa.

It was the year 2000, Life was going well. I had a beautiful wife, a beautiful 3 year old daughter, a good job and a new house. I was 24 and everything I had done had been successful, even if I had gone about things the hard way at times. Success was something I craved and without enough life experience I started making bad decisions and taking risks which ultimately have made life for my family and I much harder than they needed to be.

A steady job as an Engineer with an OK salary was not enough for me, so I left my job to set up my own business in landscape Gardening with a view to expansion and financial independence. The Business lasted for 15 months, the work was physically challenging and I became very fit. All of the jobs had gone well and I was establishing a good reputation. The problem was that I had been over ambitious and invested heavily in an expensive van, advertising and equipment. In order to compete as a 1 man outfit I could not afford to pay myself.

I decided that the best option would be to work evenings and started taxi driving, part time. Unfortunately this was also just breaking even and I could not pay myself a wage.

Needless to say working 18 hours a day and not paying myself lead to serious problems at home. My marriage fell apart and I moved out of the family home into a small rented flat. With all the stress of business, taxi driving, losing my wife etc I had a nervous breakdown.

Late at night in the Taxi, whilst alone in the car, it just happened, this is something that I never want to experience again.

I was approaching a Tee-Junction and my body just shut down, almost like being in a state of paralysis.

Fortunately there was no one around, the car coasted across the junction and came to rest against the hedge at the side of the road.

After a while, and I really don't know if it was seconds or minutes, the realisation of what was happening dawned on me. I pulled myself together, gave myself a slap in the face and drove carefully home.

I felt totally lost, so I turned to my Dad and explained the situation. He told me that the business and taxis had to go, I could earn proper money in Engineering so I should get myself a job.

I took a job as an Engineer in an automotive factory and was working long hours, 60-80 hours per week. For the first time in 10 years I was free and single, with the exception of looking after my daughter most weekends.

Weeknights were free time if work didn't drag on too late and my new found social life lead to a couple of years of night clubbing and abusing my body and generally wasting my life away.

The wages had been good but I'd done nothing to pay back any of the business debt, All I had to show for it was a bunch of blurred memories.

The 2 years hard work I had put in to this job had earned me a possible promotion to be the department manager or I could have chosen to take a more specialised role, either choice came with a good pay rise and prospects.

More bad decisions followed, it seemed that I was happy to spite myself to get back at my ex-wife… why should I work hard and earn more money, I'll only have to give it to her…?

I left my job and took a pay cut to work as a Manager in a small but growing Aerospace parts factory.

It was the summer of 2003, between these two jobs I took 3 days out to have a mini break. I took my then 6 year old daughter to Amsterdam.

We spent 2 nights in a cheap hotel, saw a lot of sights and avoided the red light district!

Whilst we were exploring the famous canals in a pedal boat, I managed to hurt my leg in a bizarre accident, my right foot slipped off the pedal and my shin hit the bulkhead of the boat quite hard leaving a significant bruise.

This injury seemed trivial to me at the time, as I had always recovered quickly from injury and illness and I didn't worry about it, after all I was young, fit, healthy and strong.

Within a week of my return however, my right leg had swollen up and I could not bend my knee properly.

This is when I first became familiar with hospital waiting rooms and blood tests. I limped into the hospital and waited.

The junior nurse took blood 5 times, with at least 8 attempts in total to find a vein. Each time there was a problem and they needed more… 'we didn't get enough blood', 'we need to do another test' and 'we lost the sample' were among the reasons.

I was so annoyed that 3 hours of my time were being wasted like this and my arms were getting sore too.

The tests for DVT came back negative and I was discharged from hospital, with pin cushions for arms, looking like a heroin addict. The nurse advised me to come back the next week if it got worse.

Next week I went back to the emergency ward at the hospital with 1 ankle, 1 'cankle' and a limp. More blood tests followed and a positive test for DVT came back.

I was sent up to a ward and a vein-o-gram was required.

This might sound like a strip-o-gram with bulging veins! The reality however is even worse! It is a procedure where dye is injected into a vein and the blood flow is viewed with an x-ray video.

My foot was so swollen that they could not find a vein, so the large needle was eventually forced in through the inside of my big toe.

All I can remember is pain like nothing else that I could have imagined, whilst 'trying to stay still'. The nurse told me afterwards that I kicked the doctor several feet across the room – (Sorry!).

After all this I was told that 'there is no blood clot, you can go home'. Which begged the question – why is my leg swollen and I can't walk properly? But there was no answer or referral back to the original doctor.

I limped out of the hospital and decided I would sort this out myself and didn't go back.

For months I limped about, taking 2-4 aspirin a day and trying to jog or walk as much as I could to keep things moving – a bad decision as it turns out.

If I had taken care at this point I would have recovered fully, however one more bad decision changed my life forever.

I had just finished rebuilding a motor bike, it was a rare 250cc race bike from Japan which was small, especially for my 6'3" frame and long legs. The petrol tank was empty as I had drained it prior to re-spray.

It was only ½ mile to the petrol station so rather than fetch a gallon of petrol in a can, I decided I could push the bike the ½ mile and fill up.

Pushing the motorbike was a struggle with the bad leg but I pushed on un-deterred. Once fuelled up, I just about managed to kick start the engine with the bad leg and got on.

I then realised that my bad leg could not bend far enough to reach the foot peg, also turning right at the junction was a problem as I my leg was sore when I tried to support the bike on the right hand side, so I decided to turn left, away from home, then go to the nearest roundabout and turn around.

My thigh ached as I was riding along, leg sticking out in front of me (in the same way that Moto-GP riders do nowadays as they approach a slow corner).

On approach to the roundabout, I thought it would be best to keep my speed up and pull out ahead of an approaching car, rather than stopping to give way, then disaster struck.

As I leaned the bike into the bend, I was busy watching where I was going and the cars that were around me, still doing 30 mph when BANG, my right foot touched to road and it was forced back, compressing the fluid in my swollen knee. The impact was so hard that lifted the back wheel of the motorbike into the air.

The pain was incredible and made the recent big toe injection feel like a 'slight scratch' and I almost blacked out. Somehow I stayed conscious with eyes like saucers, stayed on the bike and managed to continue on and ride it home.

Yet another bad decision followed as the memory of the poor treatment I had received at the hospital lead me to decide that this was another good injury for home treatment.

Again, a poor decision in hindsight, does anyone have a time machine I can borrow?

My knee was now very swollen and I had become very good at hopping around on 1 leg. I limped about like this for a year before finally seeing a doctor.

By the time I had got an MRI scan 18 months had passed and this revealed a torn ligament and crushed cartilage. Bits of damaged cartilage were hanging out of the side of my knee joint and this was causing a lot of the swelling.

After another 6 months I was finally operated on and the knee was a lot better, although any twisting would pinch what cartilage was left. After a further year of self-prescribed and administered 'physiotherapy' and careful jogging and cycling, I was able to walk almost normally.
I believe that this was the trigger for Psoriatic arthritis. My immune system may well have reacted to this damaged, swollen cartilage and activated antibodies to attack this tissue as if it were a foreign body. Whilst I cannot prove this, it seems to be a logical explanation.

Chapter 2 – The onset of Psa.

At this point I was 29, had been single for nearly 4 years.

Experience was making me realise what was important in life and I started to make more of an effort with my ex-wife and daughter.

Something just fell into place and we got back together. It took a while for things to get fully back to normal and to regain each other's trust, but we were back together as a family and nothing was going to take that away from us again.

That's when the Arthritis started to become apparent, I remember my 30th birthday well, my wife, daughter and I went camping. This is my last milestone memory of feeling 'normal'.

Shortly after this the symptoms of Arthritis developed.

I had been getting aches and pains and tried to ignore them. I thought that because I had started exercising again, maybe my body was just not ready for it.

The symptoms came on gradually and as I got used to a certain level of aches and pains it gradually got just a little bit worse week by week. It started in the soles of my feet, with a feeling like someone had been beating them with a baseball bat. I took it easy and tried to push through it.

A game of Golf with work proved to be very difficult and I could hardly walk the following day. Were my shoes to blame?

Soon, both of my Achilles tendons were swollen and I could not lift my body weight on the balls of my feet.

At the same time my lower back and neck were always aching. I thought this was a separate problem. Months passed and I put up with it as it got progressively worse.

Then one night I went to town with friends from work and had a few beers, maybe six or seven.

Whilst staggering home I noticed that my fingers were swelling up and throbbing.

My wedding ring would not come off due to the swelling so I knew it was not my imagination.

Work was getting more and more stressful as the small company I had joined was growing and my hands began swelling up over the coming weeks.

I began losing the range of movement in my fingers so that I could no longer make a fist.

Sharp pains developed in many of my finger joints and everyday tasks became very difficult.

I could no longer open jars, crisp packets or tie my laces – not for lack of trying either.

Gradually I realised that all of these problems were connected and I finally saw sense and booked an appointment with the local doctor.

Of course, I wasn't going to go in cold, I was too smart for that, wasn't I?

After a bit of internet research I had cross referenced any conditions I had.

I had patches of Psoriasis on my knees, elbows and in various other places, so I added Psoriasis into the search engine by chance and some interesting information popped up.

Psoriatic Arthritis, what's that? I thought.

I had never heard of the condition before and thought that Arthritis only happened to old people.
At the appointment with the local doctor I asked about Psoriatic Arthritis. She had never heard of this and she told me that there is no link between Psoriasis and joint pain.
I was given a prescription for pain killers and ordered me to rest for a week. Well I wasn't having any of that so I threw the prescription in the bin and went back to work.
What a waste of time that was, I thought to myself, I would be clever and sort this problem out myself.
Looking back on it now, maybe I should have done what the doctor ordered and then returned

a week later, or I should have sought a second opinion?

What I did instead was press on and try to cope with it by myself whilst the clock was ticking and more damage was being done to my joints and tendons.

By 2007, aged 31, walking from the car park to the office was almost impossible most days. I felt like a 90 year old that had fallen down the stairs. Many tendons and joints were inflamed in my fingers, wrists, elbows, shoulders, neck, back, hips knees, ankles feet and toes. Life was miserable.

We had sold our house and moved into a rented property just as the symptoms had started. Unfortunately the contract was for 12 months and we heard that the house would be sold just before the contract was going to finish.

We searched for places to rent and found a smaller bungalow near to our daughters' school, it seemed ideal.

The problem was that money was tight and friends and relatives were busy, so we hired a van and moved most of our possessions ourselves, with some help with the larger items. This house move took all of my physical and mental strength, along with 8 ibuprofen per day to help control the inflammation in so many joints and tendons.

The only thing that kept me going was the motivation to provide a home for my family, along with gritty determination not to fail.

After about 5 days of hard slog we had moved everything and tidied up the old house.

Just before my 32nd birthday, an unusual event occurred at work which taught me something else about my condition. One of the machinists was an 'ex' heroin addict and I was sure he was still using drugs.

I had warned the Directors that this was happening and that the individual should not have been taken on permanently but my advice was not heeded.

On the day in question, which was just after payday, he was staggering about at work as usual under the influence of drugs.

He went to his car for lunch and didn't come back, so one of the Directors went to his car 30 minutes later to find him sleeping it off. He was woken up and promptly sacked. I heard about this which made me quite angry.

2 minutes later, as predicted, a fight broke out in the factory involving this individual with several employees, breaking equipment and windows. One of the ladies from the factory came in and shouted 'they're fighting' so I jumped out of my office chair and ran into the factory.

OK, what's wrong with this picture?

Pain, Arthritis, limping, more pain, can hardly walk – how could I jump up and run?

The answer was adrenaline.

The problem with a big rush of adrenaline is that for a while, you feel great as if nothing can stop you, then you come down from it, but with Psoriatic arthritis there is a backlash when the adrenalin wears off the symptoms come back much, much worse for a couple of days.
That night I got home and collapsed on the sofa, exhausted. That is where I slept until the next morning.

When I woke up the Arthritis was worse than ever, I could hardly stand, but I needed to get to work so I crawled off the sofa and gradually found a way to get up on my throbbing, stinging, swollen feet and drag myself to work.
I still did not know what was affecting me as the doctor had dismissed Psoriatic Arthritis and I had taken her word for it.
I had forgotten about Psoriatic Arthritis as I battled on with a view to hopefully finding out what was causing all of my individual symptoms.

A month or two later there was no improvement and I was living on 8 ibuprofen tablets a day just to enable me to carry on as normal.

Work was totally exhausting and after a 10 hour day in the office I would come home and fall asleep, completely shattered.

The only relief I could get was having a long soak in a hot bath. This alleviated the pain and swelling for a few hours after and was absolute bliss.

I couldn't tell you how many times I fell asleep in a bath full of hot water to be woken up by the water becoming cold about an hour later, only my height prevented me from possibly drowning.

It was summer 2007 by now and I took a few days off work for a family break and was surprised at how much better I was feeling. Maybe it was my job that was causing the problem – was it the stress? Reaction to chemicals? Who knows?

As we spent a few days staying away with relatives in London, it dawned on me that I hated that job, I was so stressed and the conditions were poor.

Drastic action was required and something had to change so in a moment of madness I signed into my work computer remotely and resigned with immediate effect, by email and never went back.

I sold my motorbike to pay the bills for a month and to work out what to do next whilst we enjoyed staying in North London.

Our relatives had gone on Holiday and had allowed us to 'House sit' for a week whilst we relaxed and spent a bit of time as a family. The symptoms eased considerably during this break and I almost felt like I was back to normal.

It was 2007 and there had been severe flooding in my home town of Gloucester, which had led to power cuts and the mains waster had been off for 2 weeks.

On return to Gloucester we found that there was almost no temporary work about worth taking, so I went back to the company that I left 4 years previously and ended up getting my old job back. However, after about a month into the new - old job, all of the symptoms were back and getting worse. Any small amount of stress was triggering reactions.

For once I decided to do the right thing and went back to my new G.P. She listened to my symptoms and referred me to a Rheumatology consultant.

Chapter 3 – Finally, a diagnosis.

I went along to the appointment with a feeling that there may be hope, which I was supressing in case this turned out to be another waste of time.

The consultant was a young man, smartly dressed and enthusiastic. I remember his chinos and patterned socks very vividly. He was fairly junior and I wondered if this was a good or bad thing? Bad because of a short career and limited experience or good because of his enthusiasm.

My blood test had been negative for Rheumatoid factor. This was good news and bad news – If I didn't have Rheumatoid Arthritis then what was wrong with me?

I poured out all of my symptoms and problems to him and he listened intently. He then asked whether I had ever had a bad back or stiff neck, to which I answered yes and showed him the areas that had been an issue, more in the middle of my spine and not muscular pain.

He then asked to look at my finger nails. This puzzled me, but I held out my hands trustingly as this young doctor was inspiring me with confidence. He remarked on my pitted nails and wrote down a couple of notes. It was then that he just came out and said it:-

'You have Psoriatic Arthritis'.

I was taken aback, It was as if time had stopped for a moment, the background seemed to zoom out like an out of body experience in a film and it felt like a surreal dream. I was in disbelief, shock, relieved and I felt as though a weight had been lifted from my shoulders.
The consultant explained that he would give me an injection of a steroid (5 mls depo-medrone, intro muscular) and some leaflets on drugs called NSAIDS and DMARDS – by now I was just nodding my head and going through the motions.

It felt as if it was someone else's diagnosis that I had heard. I have never felt like this before or since.

I had been battling an unknown condition for over a year and finally I could understand the consequences and long term outlook.

The nurse prepared a syringe and gave me the injection into my left buttock. As she withdrew the needle she quickly grabbed some cotton wool and pressed it on the injection site. She apologised and said that she appeared to have caught a vein. The bleeding stopped after a minute or two and I got a plaster for my troubles. The next stop was for a series of X-Rays after which I left the hospital appointment.

I had ridden my new motorbike to the hospital, it was a cheap hack of 650cc capacity that I had bought for travelling to work and back. I rode straight back to work to make up the hours I had missed.

I remember feeling Euphoric like I could take on the world, almost like superman flying triumphantly away from another averted disaster, so much so that I went around a bend too fast and almost crashed, it was only the kerb that stopped me from leaving the road completely at 60 mph into trees and barriers, but I almost didn't care! I laughed demonically inside my crash helmet, steaming up the visor.

The walk up the 30+ steps to my office seemed rather easy and after an hour at my desk came the realisation that there was no pain.

I stood up, stretched my legs a bit and then crouched down cautiously and stood back up un aided or without holding onto something for the first time in about 3 years.

The effect of the steroid had been almost immediate, probably due to some of it getting directly into my blood stream.

The significance of the diagnosis and the success of the steroid injection then finally started to dawn on me. This isn't a dream, I thought to myself. I'm going to be cured! The thought of spending quality time with my family and friends again and knowing that I wouldn't become a burden for my long suffering wife, made me so happy and relieved that my eyes welled up and a tear ran down my face.

It should be noted that I am not an emotional person and I rarely cry, not even at funerals. The only time I had felt this good and shed a tear of joy was at the birth of my first daughter, and to be fair, a few years later again at the birth of my second daughter – but that is another, complicated story!

This emotional outpouring was also a product bottling up all of the frustration from the constant requirement for determination and struggle to carry on. I would not be beaten by this condition and the sheer effort that had been required to get on with life relatively un-aided was now being released.

In the year leading up to the diagnosis I had subconsciously written the rest of my active life off. We had already moved into a bungalow to avoid having to use stairs at home, I had given up golf and sold my golf clubs, cancelled my gym membership, given up playing guitar and generally turned into a very grumpy old man – aged 32.

But now there was light at the end of the tunnel. The steroids had worked so effectively and I felt a new sense of hope. Within a few days however, the steroids wore off and the symptoms came back even worse.

This was WAR! There was no way on this earth I would be trapped in this condition.

Psoriatic Arthritis was not going to define me! I *WAS* going to beat it!

I approached life with a new vigour and found the strength to push through the pain even more than before, because finally there was hope!

This is what is required to beat chronic illness, realise what is important, fight for it, give yourself a 100% chance and no matter what happens, never give up.

Chapter 4 – Medication & side effects.

During my treatment I was given a range of different drugs with varying effects and side effects. This is a summary of the medications I have tried.

Depo-medrone

As mentioned in chapter 2, I was injected with Depo-medrone (steroid) and given a number of X rays including my chest and spine.
The first major side effect was a big one. Although it was never attributed to any specific medication or treatment, I was told that the X-rays may have been responsible. It is also possible that the intro-muscular steroid injection that inadvertently entered my bloodstream directly my have been a factor. Either way I believe that this side effect was an aggravation of an existing issue.

What was the side effect? You ask… Well I nearly died from a Heart problem – Nothing Major!

I had woken up at about 5am on the Sunday morning 8 or 9 days after diagnosis. My wife was out working nightshift 8-8 so I was on my own and I had fallen asleep on the sofa.

I realised that I felt a bit feint and my heart was beating hard with the rhythm all over the place – (a bit like my drunken nightclub dancing!). There were intermittent flutters, followed by a pause for about two seconds then two or three beats and then a spasm etc in a random order. The condition was a form of atrial fibrillation called multifocal atrial tachycardia (MAT) – this differs from a basic arrhythmia or tachycardia as the timing between the heart chambers goes out of sync, so ones heart is working hard but pumping blood very inefficiently. This can lead to strokes or even heart attack within a few hours apparently – I didn't know any of this at the time.

So – What did I do? After about 10 minutes lying there trying to stay calm and get it to stabilise, it was persistently in spasm and fluttering etc. Slow deep breaths were not helping so I was going to fight this head on, but How???

If it wasn't responding to relaxing and lying down, I needed to give my heart some work to do, Kill or cure style! So I got up and staggered into the spare room and fired up the treadmill.

After a few minutes of trying to jog on the treadmill I was close to passing out, so 'running it off' was not an option!

Back to Plan A – I got a cup of water and returned cautiously to the sofa, with the cordless phone next to me as a precaution I put my feet up and waited.

I knew there was a chance I could go into cardiac arrest and even die, however the last few years had changed me. I was not afraid of death and I had this blasé attitude to the problem. Maybe this is a good thing, the type of feeling that some religious people get when they trust their god and resign themselves to whatever fate awaits them. My only worry was that my daughter might have to discover me on the sofa, so I focussed on staying alert and trying to regulate my heartbeat. My wife was finishing at 8:00 so at 8:05am I called her and calmly explained that I needed her to check out my heart rhythm. She rushed straight home and with a quick listen to my chest she insisted that we immediately go to the hospital emergency ward. She quickly gathered up our 10 year old daughter and helped me out to the car.

We arrived at the hospital and I walked in under my own steam – I even swung my legs over the entrance barrier to get in front of a lady limping towards the entrance with what looked like a twisted ankle. Apologies to that lady if I pushed in, but I felt my need was greater at that moment. I informed the receptionist of my predicament and she took all my details, then I proceeded to sit down, feeling more feint than ever. I had put my feet up on the chairs and a passing nurse was giving me a disapproving look (as if I was just a left over Saturday night drunk) so I told her that my heart was not right and my feet were up to ease the pressure / blood flow.

At this point the passing nurse noticed how pale I must have looked and rushed back the way she came, returning a few moments later with a senior looking doctor.

They took me straight to a bed, attached me to an ECG machine and took venal and arterial bloods. My blood oxygen saturation was about 90% - I thought that was good, but apparently anything under 98% is bad.

The doctor asked how long this episode had been going on, when I told him it was continuously for 4 hours he looked quite worried and told me that people have been known to die after a few hours in this condition.

They wheeled me into a side room on the bed, it was eerily silent with no one else about and 2 or 3 defibrillators in a row opposite to 3 empty beds.

A patch of skin about 6" by 6" was quickly shaved on my back and chest where my heart was located and they attached electrode pads.

I was given a general anaesthetic and the next thing I remember was waking about 20 minutes later, feeling OK. Well – that was easy, wasn't it? The Doctor explained that I had been given 2 shocks of DC cardio-version, front to back (not side to side as in most cases). My heart had to be stopped 2 times in order for it to start back up and regain its normal rhythm.

Now, on television dramas, these shocks are seemingly given to re start the hearts of patients that had flat lined due to apparent heart attacks. The patients chest usually goes up and down and then usually remains silent… this is what I imagined had happened to me.

In reality however, it is a completely different story. The reason I was taken around to a side room for this procedure became clear when I spoke to my wife shortly after being discharged.

She and my daughter had been in the room, on the other side of the drawn curtains. She recalled what had happened whilst I was out under anaesthetic.

I could see that she had been traumatised, along with my poor little girl. I then looked at my daughter and realised she had been crying, my wife explained why.

The effect of the DC Cardio-version was much more graphic than the televised shocks. As the doctor applied each shock I had apparently let out a traumatic sound, the type you might imagine someone making whilst having a leg or arm ripped off in a horror film.

This was combined with the sound of 220 pounds of me crashing around on the trolley.

They must have thought that I was going to die and I wish they had not had to witness such an event.

Fortunately I was OK and typically Blasé about the whole affair.

Rolling into work at 7:30 am the next day, I showed off the shaved squares and burn marks on my chest and back and joked that it would take more than having my heart stopped and restarted to keep me out of work!

My colleagues were suitably concerned and made sure that I had a relatively easy couple of days.

The following Sunday, however, I woke up with the same problem – this time I avoided the treadmill! My wife came back from another 12 hour nightshift and again rushed me into hospital. This time the doctors connected me to a drip and administered a strong beta blocker intravenously, which sorted the problem out within about 15 minutes. I was then prescribed oral beta blockers called Bisoprolol, which I took for 6 months before many tests revealed that I was OK. Fortunately I have only ever had two further events, with a 45 minute episode that stopped as I reached hospital (typical) and another 15 minute episode. I occasionally get the odd missed beat following all of this, however it has not stopped me from living my life and pushing hard, especially when cycling up hills – more details of cycling to follow.

I returned to the rheumatology consultant 3 months later and was given another shot of depo-medrone steroid, this time without incident. This took 2-3 days for the benefit to be felt as per the design and the benefits were much more subtle, however after a month the symptoms were coming back harder, as if it was a post – steroidal backlash.

During this appointment, I discussed the next stage of medication.

The leaflets that the consultant gave me at the first appointment had been left on the side waiting for a moment of peace so that I could read them carefully. The reading had not been good.

There were two types of disease-modifying anti-rheumatic drug (DMARD) that I could try, called Methotrexate and Sulphasalazine.

Methotrexate

Methotrexate was an early Chemotherapy drug, however the doses would be much smaller than those used to treat cancer. This was taken once per week in tablet form.
I chose to start on Methotrexate. I liked the idea of only having to remember to take the tablets once a week as I am usually quite busy and pre occupied. The preferred day was Friday after work.
4 tablets were taken each Friday evening and by Saturday morning I would usually feel pretty rough, cold, shivery and tired – prompting a 'siesta' style nap most weekends.
However my symptoms started to improve slightly and the side effects lessened as I got used to the drugs, so I had a glimmer of hope that this would work for me.
After 3 months my condition was bearable. Getting out of bed my feet were painful at first but

after gentle stretching and walking carefully they would free up.

I could make a fist now, however there was a stiffness in my hands that has never fully gone away, and my wedding ring still did not fit due to the swelling.

Every cloud has a silver lining, as they say and the finger swelling was a bonus because I have average sized hands, but at 6'3", they look relatively small – the sausage fingers took care of that!

Methotrexate alone was not enough and I was taking a non steroidal anti inflammatory drug (NSAID) called Diclofenac sodium.

This combination seemed to work OK for about 6 months but then it started to loose it's effectiveness as my immune system started to find ways around this medication.

The next problem with methotrexate is the warning regarding conceiving children. If one wants to conceive, then the drugs must be out of your system for 6 months.

We had tried for another child prior to medication but had been unsuccessful, mainly due to stress. However when I was taking Methotrexate we forgot to use contraception just once and sure enough, about 6 weeks later we realised that we were 'expecting'.

This was devastating news as we were sure that we would need an abortion. We booked an emergency appointment with the doctor to discuss what to do, but surprisingly she was positive and booked us in for a scan and advised my wife to start taking folic acid. We had many extra tests and scans and worried the whole time that our child could have been affected in some way.

Please, please, please be careful with contraception when taking Methotrexate and the other DMARD's. The stress and worry were immense and many tears were shed.

We were very lucky and in September 2009 I became a dad again to a perfect little girl.

Sulphasalazine

My consultant had changed and the new doctor prescribed Sulphasalazine.
Sulphasalazine was a newer DMARD which required taking tablets regularly, starting at one 500mg tablet Once Daily to four tablets per day.
A word of warning (especially to the men reading this) – the brand of Sulphasalazine that I was using had a strong yellow colour which was filtered out by my kidneys and made my urine bright orange. This stained really badly and a drop on the toilet seat would leave a stubborn stain within seconds.
Furthermore if standing at a urinal I became quite self conscious… No - nothing to do with 'size envy' - but due to the incredibly bright orange colour of the urine I was passing!
To bridge the gap between medications, I was given a 28 day supply of oral steroids called Prednisolone. These worked exceptionally well

and it is a shame that these cannot be taken long term.

Sulphasalazine seemed to work OK and again my symptoms improved for 6 months, enough to make life bearable, however I still struggled with grip and could not run. In order to make improvements I changed the NSAID from Diclofenac to Naproxen.

Again with this combination things went well for a few months but then they started to loose effectiveness.

Although the severity of the individual joint and tendon inflammation was improved, the condition was by now spreading.

My shoulders, elbows and neck were getting stiff and problematic, including a worrying click in my neck when turning my head.

The Naproxen was having other side effects that were intangible, but it seemed to make me angry. After a few months of getting more and more intolerant of people around me I found myself in a spot of road rage.

To cut a long story short, I was taking my mother to a local department store in her car. She was in need of 2 hip replacements so she had a disabled badge. I had parked on the side of the road waiting for a disabled space to become free. My mother had walked into the store alone and I was waiting for an elderly couple taking a long time to get into their car, so that I could park and go in to help mum with her shopping.

Another driver pulled up behind me, then realised I was waiting and made a bit of a drama about having to drive around our car. They then turned around and drove back past, with the driver visibly mouthing complaints at me for waiting there.

Now normally, I would have smiled back or even chuckled a little bit at this, but with the Naproxen induced rage I flung the door open and jumped out of the car, waving my arms about angrily and shouting something like *'Come on then, get out of your 'effing car, I'll 'effing Batter you, you twat!!!'* …etc. – you get the point.

It was lunchtime on a Saturday in busy town centre. Lots of people were looking, mostly shocked. Oops.

At this point I had a really good think. Why was I so angry and irritated? It seemed that the Naproxen was doing this to me, making my Psoriasis flare up too and making me feel particularly irritated.

My poor wife and daughter had put up with this moodiness to a certain extent, but it was not worth it for the grief I was causing them, and I certainly didn't want to get involved in any rage induced fights in town.

I stopped taking Naproxen and reverted to plain old trusted store brand Ibuprofen – this seemed to work OK and I felt psychologically more normal after a week or two.

12 months of Sulphasalazine and the effectiveness was receding and I needed to try something else.

Leflunomide

My third consultant recommended a newly available DMARD called Leflunomide, or commonly known as a trade mark 'Arava'. Initially 10 mg per day – this progressed to 20 mg per day and was the most effective of the three DMARDS for me. I used this for 2 years (2009-2011) with little or no side effects and it remained fairly effective for the entire duration.
The Ibuprofen reliance was minimised too. This was a good thing as all of these tablets were playing havoc with my stomach. A reduced amount of Ibuprofen and one Leflunomide tablet per day were less traumatic on my stomach than the previous medications and I was no longer getting regular indigestion and heartburn.
I would highly recommend trying Leflunomide (Arava) as it was the most effective chemical DMARD in my case.
However, none of the DMARDs stopped the disease spreading.

Humira (adalimumab)

When visiting my consultant, who this time happened to be the original young enthusiastic chap I had seen with the chinos and golf style socks, I explained that I had been through Methotrexate and Sulphasalazine with limited success. The Leflunomide, which I had been taking at this point for 18 months, was working well to supress the severity of my symptoms but more joints and tendons were becoming affected as time passed.

The consultant asked me that considering I was feeling better now, had I at all considered going back to work?

I told him It had been tough and painful, but I hadn't had a single day off work through illness for 8 years.

He looked surprised and commended me on this. Most people he was treating had given up on work and life and were focussing on pain relief and rest.

Now I need to be clear that I am in no way implying that if anyone with Arthritis of any kind is no longer working that that is a bad thing. We are all different. For me, I have a high pain threshold and a very strong motivation to be at work, providing for my family – it is what drives me.

We all have different symptoms, pain thresholds, motivation and of course, jobs. I was lucky that my job was varied and I could be at my desk or walking around a factory. When my hands were particularly bad I could get one of my colleagues to help with things such as lifting or making adjustments to equipment etc.

The lesson here is that no matter how bad you feel as a result of your arthritis, don't give up on life. You MUST cling to what ever it is that is important to you and keep on enjoying life as much as possible. You never know what may happen next and things can get better, especially if you stay mobile.

Back to the medication – the consultant told me that based on my age, 35 at the time, and the fact that I was working and also quite badly affected, that I could qualify for 'anti TNF alpha' treatment funding.

I was booked in for an appointment with the Rheumatology nurse for examination. If I recall correctly there were 71 joints on her chart, of which 57 were inflamed or painful. I only needed at least 9 to qualify.

The next treatment was called Humira (or adalimumab), which was based on a monoclonal human antibody. As far as I can tell, these cloned antibodies get into one's bloodstream and provide a sacrificial target for those antibodies which are targeting one's connective tissue.

Once I had been approved, a nurse came to my home to show me how to inject myself with the Humira.

I pinched an area of skin on my abdomen, pressed the pen firmly in place and pressed the button. Bang! The spring loaded needle fired into my skin and injected the drug.

If you have ever had a wasp sting, that is what this feels like… like getting an angry wasp and thrusting its sting into your belly, then holding it there whilst counting for 10 seconds.

Apart from the stinging it was not that exciting. The nurse said it would take 4-6 weeks until I notice a difference.

The next day I woke up and got out of bed and walked to the bathroom. No pain!!! (well, at least a lot less that I was by now used to). This was great, was I dreaming? Hell no! just like with the depo-medrone steroids I felt almost normal.

This was not a placebo effect. I was told this may take many weeks to work, if at all and I was not expecting any sort of effect that day. For some reason Humira was working very well straight away.

The range of motion in my fingers was improving and I could crouch again. I stopped taking Ibuprofen straight away and have not needed to go back to taking it since.

A word of caution. Years of reduced physical activity due to arthritis can lead to weakening of your muscles, tendons and joints. I was so excited about this that I was bouncing around, lifting heavy things and getting up to all sorts of mischief. It is best to approach the good days with a cautious and careful approach and to build up activity levels slowly.

I lifted one side of a large metal container at work, weighing over 100 kg total (why? – because I could!) and promptly hurt my back.

I also managed to tear my upper calf muscle very badly, requiring more visits to hospital to check why my leg was swollen.

Fortunately technology had moved on since the previous blood clot scare and they used ultrasound rather than a long needle to inject die into your blood... phew!

I find that for the last few days before each injection of Humira in the 2 week cycle, my feet and hands start to flare up a bit, reminding me that I have Psoriatic Arthritis and to take care, however just after each injection, the symptoms die down significantly. The other benefit is that my Psoriasis has almost completely cleared up, with the exception of a little stubborn bit on each knee.

The effect that Humira has had on my Quality of life is incredible and I would describe this as life changing! I felt like I had been given a second chance in life. It was mid 2011 and 2012 was going to be a great year!!!

Chapter 5 – 2012, what a year!

By chance, I had found a really good job advertised in a professional magazine. I left my stressful job in the troubled automotive industry and became an auditor for a large company that operates power stations in the UK.

It was September 2011, the 3 months of Humira had started to work well and I was now enjoying cycling to work as it was now much less painful. Furthermore, my new job was proving to be a lot less stressful and I was able to focus on one job at a time rather than getting bombarded with multiple urgent problems at the same time as with my old job.

I was moved to a desk sitting next to a keen cyclist, who told me about a cycling club after work that could be interesting.

My fitness level was pretty poor even though I had continued to cycle 5 miles each way to work (not by choice, but for financial reasons). Humira had made cycling bearable again, even slightly enjoyable!

My first ride out with the club was with the slower of the two groups, called the 'leisure ride'. We took a slightly shorter route than the fast group and I thought we were going well. Riding with others was new to me and I was starting to enjoy the social side of cycling.

About 15 miles into the ride, going up a gentle incline I was carrying about 14 mph near the front of the pack on my trusty hybrid bike. Then the fast group, having completed a few extra miles of diversion, flew past on their road bikes and lycra outfits as if we were standing still.

This inspired me, I wanted to go fast with those guys, but could I?

I immediately went out and purchased a road bike and some lycra clothing to match.

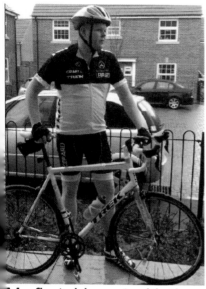

My first ride out with the new gear.

Those few rides out in October 2011 inspired me to push myself and improve. Up until then I had been in damage limitation mode, now I could start to push myself again and attempt to be at least mildly competitive. With this hope came a new found self-esteem and confidence.

Winter set in and the road bike went into storage whilst the old hybrid took the brunt of the winter. Running was still off limits, even though short jogs of up to 50 metres were becoming possible. But with cycling I had a chance to be physically equal to my peers and I was able to join in and feel 'normal'. I couldn't wait for the spring to come along with the evening club rides.

My confidence was building. Work was going well and I could cycle 25 miles at a decent pace. In the spring I went out for a drink with an old friend from school days for a bit of a catch up. He had taken up running a few years prior to this and lost a significant amount of weight. However, running was tough and in order to train without having as much impact on his knees and feet he had also taken up cycling.

I talked about the cycling club at work and my new road bike. He told me that he was doing a charity bike ride and insisted that I should join him.

I didn't really have a choice in the matter so I agreed and went home. Then it dawned on me, I had no Idea what the charity was or what distance was involved.

What had I signed up for? Could I do it?

I emailed my friend a few days later and asked for more details, but after pressing send I thought about the consequences of either decision, for or against. Could I back out and use arthritis as an excuse?

Of course I couldn't! I am too determined and maybe too stupid to give in!

It was March 2012 and there were 3 months until the ride. The charity involved was there to help local youth get assistance with going from welfare into gainful employment.

The charity was not so important now, although I must admit that I had secretly hoped for a moment that it had been something pointless like 'save the lesser spotted stick insect' so I could make my excuses, but on reflection how would I feel if I didn't give it a try. Giving up is easy at the time but the effects can be lasting and I didn't want to spend precious time wondering what if? What was important was that I was going to drag myself up from a couch potato lazy cyclist to a respectable level where I could feel like I had achieved something and do a bit of living for a change. I was fed up of years of just existing.

So what sort of ride would it be? The route went between the rugby grounds of Bristol, Bath, Gloucester and back to Bristol, taking in the beautiful Cotswold hills over a distance of 100 miles.

100 MILES!!!!! Cotswold Hills!!!!

My Gosh! could I go that far??? There was only one way to find out.

Training rides commenced in March. The first was with some other friends over a distance of about 45 miles.
My thighs were burning, calves aching, wrists elbows and shoulders all ached and I had to stop half way up the longest hill and walk, whilst completely out of breath and energy, but I eventually got back on the bike and pushed on.
The next weekend I did 54 miles. Again it was hard work and everything hurt, both during and for days after.
I now had a target to focus on, I couldn't and wouldn't fail the challenge and the pain didn't matter.
The next ride, two weeks later was with the friend that had roped me into this crazy challenge. We rode and rode out into the countryside.

Again I had to get off and walk on the steepest bit of biggest hill, but I managed to get back on and pedal on to the top.

My friend was significantly fitter than I was and I didn't want to hold him up. After 64 miles my quadriceps started to cramp badly and I was close to giving up.

Nevertheless, I had to finish this ride and we eventually reached my friends' house after a painful 72 miles.

As we approached his home and whilst freewheeling down a slight hill, I tried to take my hands off the handle bars only to find my fingers were seized and the pain in my wrists almost stopped me from pulling my fingers free.

Once I got my hands off I tried to straighten my arms one at a time but my elbows had also seized. I gradually stretched my joints out and tried to ease the stiffness in my neck. Was it worth this much pain and suffering? Of course it was, I was out doing what I would otherwise be enjoying so why let a bit of pain stop me. I smiled to myself and felt a sense of some achievement and pedalled slowly up the last little hill to my friends' house.

He kindly gave me a lift home in his car as I couldn't possibly make it the last 10 miles home, more to do with poor fitness than the pain, I think the technical name for the condition is 'jelly legs'! My body was wrecked and I had started to shiver with exhaustion, but as we drove back to my house I had a sense of elation, achievement and triumph.

I was sticking two fingers up at Psoriatic Arthritis and giving it a damn good fight. Ok so I was walking like John Wayne but in my mind I was Winning!

More training rides with work followed and I could now go out alone and push myself a little harder each time and motivate myself to go 50,60 or even 70 miles at a good pace.

Whilst discussing the charity ride at work, a colleague told me that there was a team of cyclists planning to ride for charity from Paris to London.

Of course I thought 'I can do that'! it was only 70 miles a day for 3 days, easy-peasy eh?

I immediately applied to participate but unfortunately for me the ride was oversubscribed so I could not get in.

I went about my work with a slight sense of disappointment, however I was not alone and some other fellow excluded cyclists in my department were talking about arranging a similar charity ride. I jumped at the chance, but again would I be able to do it?

It was 6 weeks until the 100 mile charity ride and I could ride 70 miles in one go, but needed a couple of days recovery before getting back on the bike.

100 miles would be hard, but at least I could rest afterwards. Several days riding in a row would be an altogether tougher challenge.

I need to acknowledge that my wife had been very accommodating and understanding about my new found hobby. Many weekends were spent working on the bike and training, whilst she stayed at home with the kids.

With a 100 mile charity bike ride looming in June, I signed up for the work charity ride. The date clashed with our 15th wedding anniversary and again I have to give praise to my wife for giving her blessing for me to take part.

The route was decided and it would be a longer route than the alternative Paris to London ride that we had missed, we were going to go one better than that.

The plan was day 1, Gloucester-Guildford, day 2 Guildford-Folkestone, channel tunnel then across Calais, Day 3 Calais to Amiens and day 4 Amiens to Paris.

Well, first things first, I had to find out if I could even complete 100 miles in one day and then how would I feel the day after?

The day of the Bristol 100 mile ride came quickly and I found myself cycling out of the car park facing the unknown.

Bristol to Bath was fairly straight forward and flat. After a quick regroup, drink and toilet stop, we had pictures taken then we began the ascent up box hill. Other cyclists came past me and my friend had disappeared off in front.

I was cycling at a steady 7 mph and recent experience had taught me not to try to keep up but to go at my own pace, so I settled into a steady rhythm that I could sustain.

Surprisingly though, I started to pass some of the keen cyclists who had previously overtaken me. I had a steady ride all the way to the top without stopping.

I made it and I wasn't in last place!

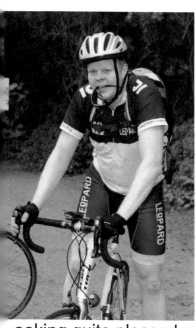

Looking quite pleased with myself at the top of box hill!

I was relieved that I was not the slowest in our group as we pressed on. The last hill before Gloucester was too much for me, about 600 feet of climbing and around 15-20% gradient. Along with a few others I had to get off and push the last and steepest 50 metres.

Lots of joints and tendons were beginning to ache now, there had been more hills than I was really used to doing during training. Should I stop off and go home which was nearby, said the little nagging voice of doubt and self-pity… I would never forgive myself so no, and especially since I had been sponsored for about £100.

Sometimes it is good to commit to challenges like this because that extra pressure of not letting down sponsors or peers can help you to find the strength you need to carry on.

After a quick lunch stop in Gloucester we pressed on for Bristol. Unfortunately a few of us took the wrong route in the confusion and took a fairly flat and direct main road, meaning that we missed a final big hill and a few miles off the distance, but with 97.2 miles on the clock in 9 hours and an average rolling speed of 13.3mph I was fairly pleased with myself.

I had kept up with the other cyclists and felt good. Surprisingly the arthritis was not giving me any significant pains.

Perhaps this was due to training, or was it the endorphins that I had released from completing a team activity. Perhaps it was both?

Gloucester to Paris – 410 miles in 4 days.

A few weeks later and the big day had arrived. As a team of twelve mixed ability cyclists from work we were going to cycle all the way to Paris. When I say mixed ability I mean I was slower than at least 9 of the guys and the best rider was aseasoned ex time trial competitor that could cover 180 miles per day with no bother.
I was quietly confident though and I had no fears about covering the distance at the group speed required.
Day one was familiar territory, 100 miles in one day, except my neck, shoulders and back were very sore, much worse than on any of the training rides, but I soldiered on regardless. It wasn't until 60 miles into the ride when we stopped for lunch that I realised the cause was my new helmet, purchased the day before the ride - it had a peak attached to the front of it that meant I had to bend my neck a few degrees further than before to see where I was going. I

ripped the blasted thing off and threw it in the bin, but it was too late and I would have neck ache for the rest of the trip. It rained almost all the way to Guildford and after a few wrong turns we ended up covering 110 miles. Between us we had fixed 8 punctures and the journey had taken 11 hours.

Soaking wet and cold we cleaned up in our hotel rooms and got ready for a late dinner.

I worried about the effects on my arthritis, as cold and damp conditions seemed to make them flare up. So I had a nice hot shower to mitigate against the effects that the cold may have had and to relieve my neck ache.

The next day would be the biggest challenge. We had to get 91 miles to Folkestone by 2 pm to get onto the Eurotunnel cycle transport we had booked, on top of this it would be the first time I had attempted two days of distance riding back to back.

I joined a group of cyclists of similar stature and ability to me and the four of us left the hotel first at 7:30am to allow enough time and get ahead of the faster riders that would set off just after 8:00am.

I was very conscious of the aches and pains from the previous day's efforts, but the aches soon eased off to manageable levels as we got going. I focussed on the task in hand, getting to Folkestone on time to catch the euro tunnel crossing.

Fortunately we had a bit of sunshine and a slight tailwind. Despite a small diversion adding 4 miles onto the journey we pressed on working as a team to share the load.

Then I hit a problem, in the shape of a pot hole. It was at the bottom of a valley and I was doing about 40 miles per hour down the hill, I noticed a defect in the road which was covering most of the lane width and I couldn't go around it. My instinctive reaction was to try to hop over it. I managed to clear it with the front wheel but the back wheel came down hard on the far edge of the pothole. The impact was so violent that my full water bottle flew out of the secure bottle mount, my left foot had been at bottom stroke and the pedal cleat had unclipped due to the impact, sending my left foot onto the road and back up into the bike frame, right on my aching Achilles tendon.

I stayed in control of the bike and, as if I was Luke Skywalker using the force, manage to kick the airborne water bottle through the frame with my flailing left foot and catch it with my right hand and neatly re holster it, all within about 1 second. Despite almost fully qualifying as a Jedi for my skills, I suffered with a bruise to my heel and my new rear wheel had a 15 mm buckle in it.

Never mind – I nursed it 10 miles to our lunch stop and got my tools out of the support van. After a couple of minutes of adjustment the buckle was minimised and the spoke tensions were back within acceptable, self-perceived limits.

Any Aches, pains and injuries were pushed to the back of my mind as we focussed on pressing on to Folkestone and the task in hand, getting to the terminal in time.

The 95 miles were completed by 2:10 pm and a well-deserved pint of lager was had by all. I joined in and had a pint of Lager too, despite knowing that lager triggers my arthritis to flare up.

We crossed into France with no problems, with the exception of trying not to seize up from sitting down for an hour, so I got up and started stretching gently – legs, arms, hips, neck. I'm not sure what the other passengers must have thought, seeing a big bloke in lycra stretching about like a rubbish Yoga student. We were dropped off near the terminal in a convenient French motorway service station car park and cycled the last few miles to the hotel in Calais, 99 miles in total.

The next two days cycling through the countryside of northern France were fantastic, with the exception of being incredibly saddle sore and not wanting to sit down.

The Arthritis was behaving remarkably well now as my body adjusted to doing 8 hours of physical exercise every day. As long as I took care to stretch and warm up before getting back on the bike things were OK.

I was in the slower of the two groups but we were not hanging around – averaging 15-16 mph.

We rolled into Paris around 5 pm on day 4 and met the faster group at the bottom of the Eiffel tower.

We made it! and we had raised £10,000 for Paralympics GB.

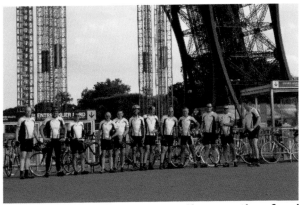

Under the Eiffel tower, I'm on the far left.

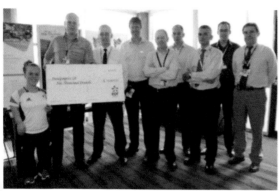

Presenting our cheque to Ellie Simmonds

Now I had the bug. Cycling long distances was normal business. For a couple of months after the Paris trip I was fitter than ever and easily able to keep up at the front of the groups when out cycling with friends. Psa was no longer a barrier or a problem, it was just there reminding me that I had a condition, but it was kept at the back of my mind and not allowed to dominate my thoughts.

I entered one final 100 mile ride, this time a sportive.

This was in October 2012 and was from Cirencester across the Cotswolds around Broadway and back to Cirencester.

There were some big hills, at least by my standards, with three 700 foot climbs en-route.

I practiced hills at every opportunity and trained to be able to stand up and go up any gradient that I was going to face.

This time I was overtaking others on the hills and waiting at the top for my friends.

For me I had won this battle against Psa.

However I am painfully aware that the War is still on-going. Psoriatic Arthritis is not going away and I will continue to fight it for as long as I live.

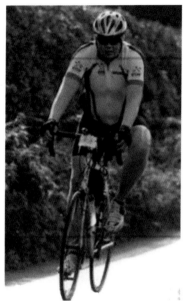

The last big ride for 2012.

Chapter 6 – Life's what you make it!

In 2012 I feel like I have really lived. It's been a struggle but with the help of the National Health Service, Humira, a ton of self-belief, motivation and determination, I have been able to take on challenges and participate in events that I could have easily stood by and watched other people doing.

My new focus is on spending time with my family. They have let me spend precious time and money chasing my dreams in 2012 and now I must give this back.

The lesson I have learned is simple. Yes, make things happen and fill your life with experiences and challenges, but remember what it is that you really want to achieve.

No one can live your life for you, you have to take control and commit to whatever it is that you want to do with your life.

And remember, no matter how bad it gets, there is always someone out there in a worse situation.

It is very easy to think, why me? or to feel sorry for yourself. I have been there and in the face of adversity felt that I had been dealt a bad hand of cards.

I have found that it is better to focus on what you can do and be grateful for what you have.

If you accept that there will be compromise, you can move forward and live life.

In my case, my fingers are less nimble and I can't play 6 string guitar properly, but I have now changed to 4 string bass which has enabled me to continue to play music and exercise my hands.

I can no longer play football or play golf, but I have found cycling. I ache in the morning but I am grateful for having all of my limbs in working order.

Even simple things like being grateful for loved ones around you or even for basics like beans on toast or a nice cup of tea. Take time to appreciate the good things in life.

Focus on the positives and the future and you WILL be able to overcome almost any obstacle.

Life's what you make it!

Chapter 7 – <u>My tips for controlling Psa</u>

These are my tips for controlling Psa based on personal experience, in the areas of exercise, food, drink, supplements, medication and lifestyle.

Exercise – do as much regular exercise as possible and stretch at every practical opportunity, you will retain flexibility and range of motion for much longer if you stay active. Even as I write this I'm having to stretch out my fingers every 15 minutes or so, then roll my shoulders, flex my neck and back just to stop them from seizing up… Cycling, walking and yoga are all good and the more regularly you take exercise the easier it will become, even if it is hard at first. Of course you need to know your limits and build up gradually, but make sure that Psa does not become an excuse not to do any exercise.

Food – Try to eat oily fish regularly, such as salmon or pilchards. Your joints need all the help they can get. Avoid particularly acidic foods and too much red meat. An interesting meat to try is goat. When your body digests goat meat it needs to produce an alkali, whereas other red meats require the production of acid to digest.

Drink – avoid caffeine and alcohol, these things make my symptoms flare up. Stay hydrated. Water and herbal tea are good.

Supplements – I take Vitamin D3, K2, L-arginine, Iron and Glucosamine on a regular basis. These seem to help repair the extra wear and tear that Psa inflicts on our joints and tendons.

Medication – try to get the best medical care. Make sure that your rheumatologists are aware off all your symptoms. But most importantly, make sure that you take medication on time and do what they tell you to do.

With Methotrexate it is important to plan when you intend to take it. I chose Friday evening so that I could use Saturdays to get through the side effects, without affecting work and having the knowledge that I didn't have to drive anywhere. Humira also requires careful planning. I have also set this up for every other Friday. This caused an issue when we cycled to France, because I would be abroad when the injection was due, however it needs to be kept refrigerated at all times. I brought the previous weeks injection forward to a Thursday morning and then the last one before the trip was injected on the Tuesday night before we departed, to ensure that I would get the maximum benefit from the injection. Humira should be taken out of the fridge and injected around 15 minutes later.

The colder it is the more it stings, however I left one out by accident for 2 hours. It was less painful to inject but it had very little effect and after another 2 weeks I was ready for another injection with multiple flare ups. 30 minutes is the longest it can be left out of the fridge for before effectiveness starts to reduce.

Some people also take a natural approach to treating Psa. Before getting onto medication I tried various ways of controlling it with diet and herbal remedies – it was then that lifestyle generally made the biggest difference.

I have no advice on what alternative therapies to take. My only recommendation is to try one thing at a time and give it a chance to work. Whenever I have tried different things, I have been impatient and changed three or more foods, medications or lifestyle choices and been left wondering which one had made me feel better! Remember it is a long term experiment so it is important to take time to ensure that you get the right result.

Lifestyle – It is important to keep stress at a low level. Everyone has problems in life but try to minimise stress where possible. There is a direct link between stress and activity of Psoriatic Arthritis.

Stay warm too. I used to walk around in a tee shirt, even if it was snowing. Keeping warm seems to alleviate the symptoms so I wear a decent coat to work and make sure that the heating is always on in the house.

My Motorbike also stays in the Garage during winter nowadays and I drive the car to work as much as possible.

When making changes to lifestyle, again try to change one thing at a time and note the results before trying another new thing.

Always stay positive. Others are in the same boat, you're not alone and you can beat Psoriatic Arthritis. The symptoms may still exist and you may have to compromise what you do, but you can still achieve great things.

Set realistic goals and write them down, with a timescale, better still join in with group or charity events if you need an extra push to find the strength to carry on.

Remember that pain is a signal to your brain telling you that your body is in distress. Use it to monitor your condition but learn to control it instead of letting pain control you.

Never, ever let yourself feel like a victim, or you will become one.

Most of all enjoy life. You only get one lifetime so don't let this condition or anything else destroy your precious time on this earth.

Good luck and be strong!

Trevor.

Acknowledgements

Special thanks to:

The National Health Service, UK

Gloucester Royal Hospital, Rheumatology

And a special thank you to my wife Paulette, you are my Rock!

Further resources:

www.Papaa.org

http://www.paralympics.org.uk/

Printed in Great Britain
by Amazon